DIABETIC SNACKS AND DESSERTS

Cookbook

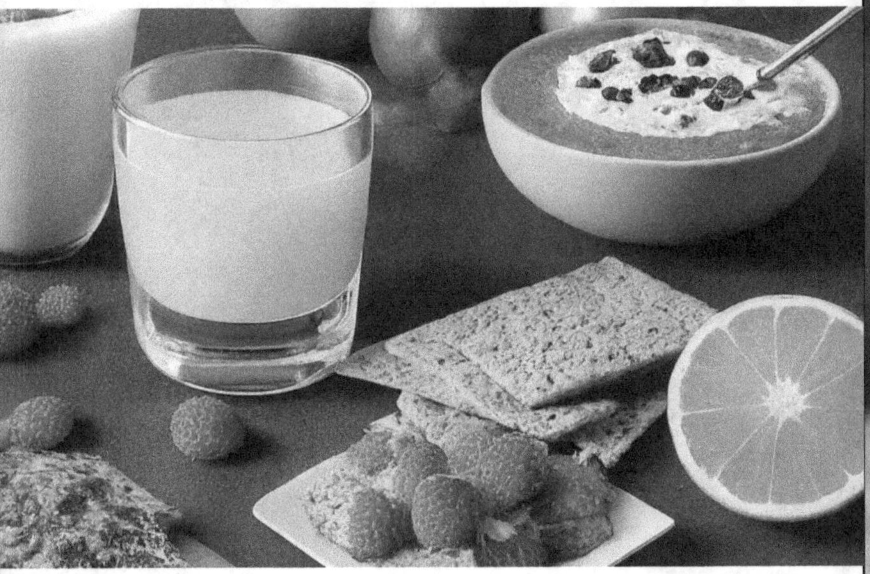

365 Days of Delicious Low-Carb, Low-Calorie, High Protein and Zero Sugar recipes for Type 1, Type 2, Gestational and Pre-Diabetic Lifestyle

Avery Stoneheart

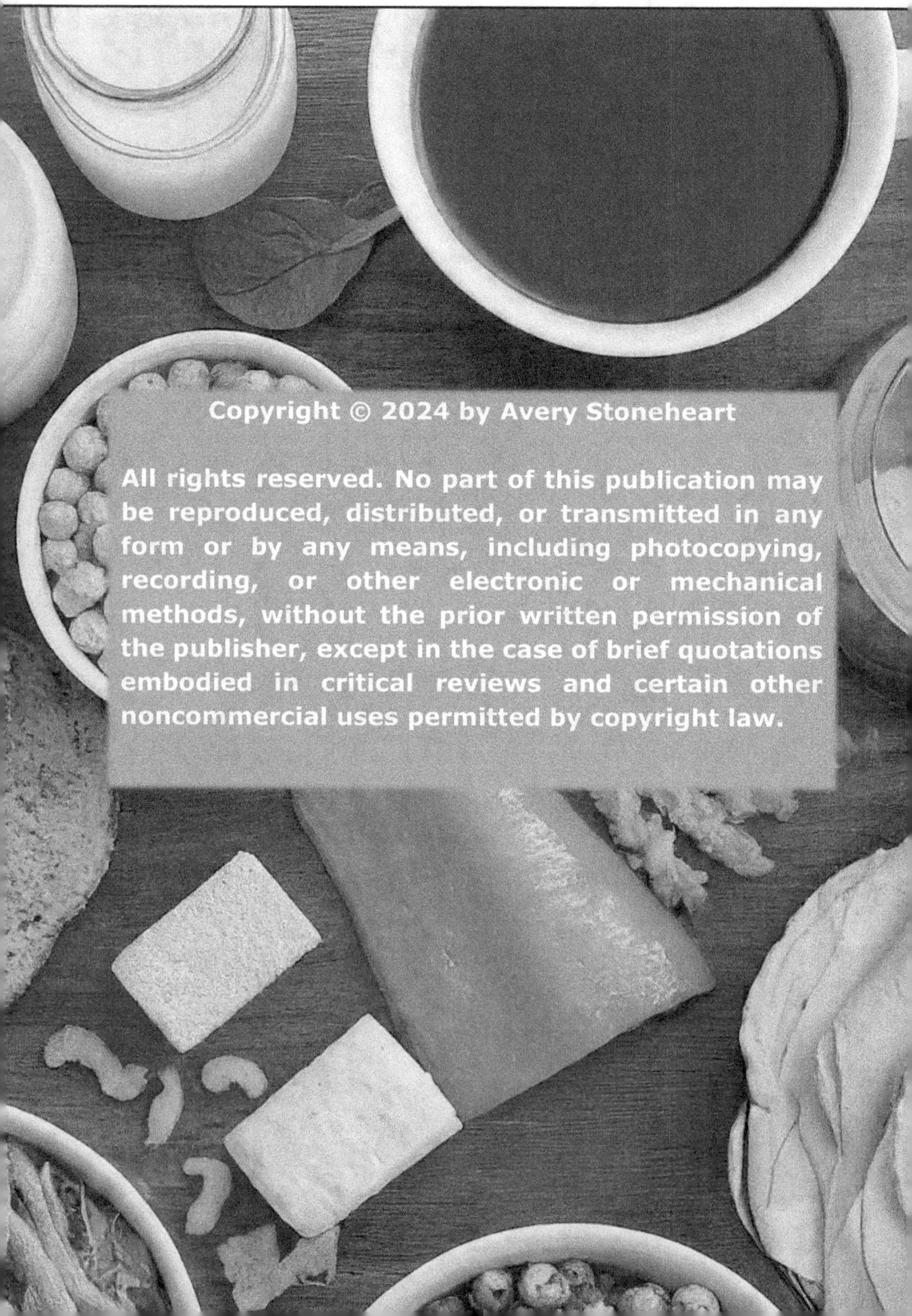

Contents

Introduction

My Story

My passion for nutrition isn't just a career path; it's a way of life. For three decades, I've stood shoulder-to-shoulder with clients and watched the transformative power of food. My expertise took a profoundly personal turn when a close family member was diagnosed with diabetes. Suddenly, the charts and textbooks turned into daily choices, meals meticulously planned, and a shared triumph over what at first felt like a monumental challenge. With every client facing diabetes, that experience resonates and drives me to make their journey easier, tastier, and more triumphant.

Diabetes & The Power of Nutrition

Whether you're living with Type 1, Type 2, gestational, or even pre-diabetes, one thing holds true: what you eat matters! It's far more than just avoiding sugar. Diabetes management through food is a symphony – balancing carbohydrates for steady energy, incorporating fiber to slow digestion, and understanding how fats play their part. Don't worry, we'll unravel all these and more!

Snacks & Desserts Reimagined

Let's shatter a myth right now: diabetes and deliciousness are NOT enemies! Yes, a diabetes-friendly diet needs adjustments, but bland

and boring are definitely off the menu. Think luscious textures, satisfying flavors, and treats that work *with* your goals, not against them. From vibrant snacks to sweet indulgences, get ready to rediscover the joy of eating— guilt-free!

My Promise to You

This book isn't just a collection of recipes, and I'm not just another voice dispensing information. Think of me as your experienced and enthusiastic guide in the kitchen. We'll explore ingredients, build confidence, and prove that living well with diabetes is absolutely attainable...and undeniably delicious!

Let's Get Cooking!

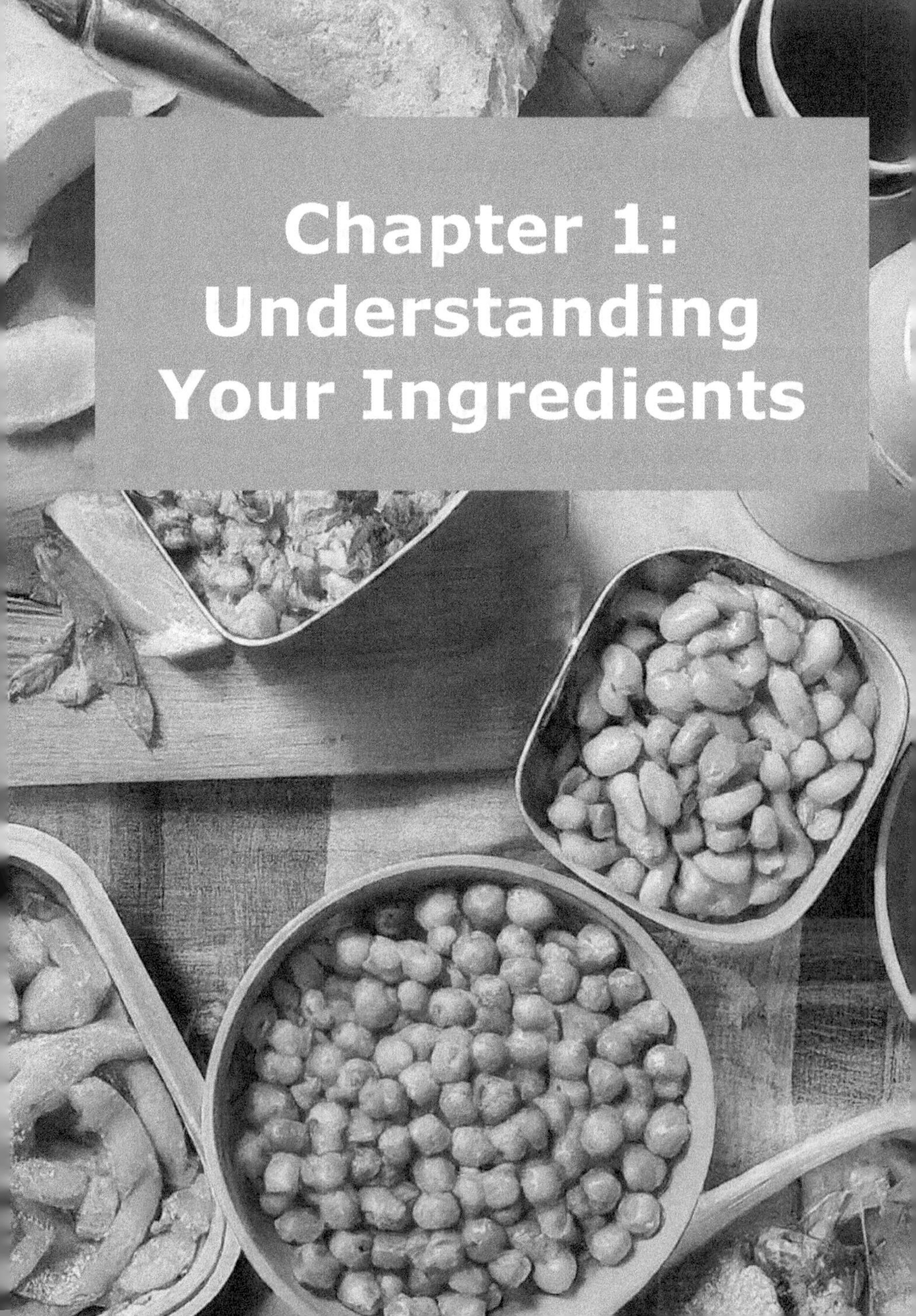
Chapter 1:
Understanding
Your Ingredients

The kitchen can be a battleground when you're managing diabetes. Familiar ingredients might suddenly seem questionable! This chapter takes the stress out of your pantry and empowers you to whip up snacks and desserts that are as delicious as they are supportive of your blood sugar goals.

Sweet Substitutions: A Sugar-Smart Toolkit

The biggest worry: replacing the sweetness sugar provides. Let's break it down into the natural and artificial camps:

1. **Nature's Helpers:** Honey, maple syrup, agave – yes, they're "natural," but they impact blood sugar just like table sugar. Yet, used *sparingly,* they add depth of flavor. You'll learn to balance them with other tactics.

2. **Artificial Sweeteners:** Aspartame, saccharin, etc. offer sweetness with negligible calories and blood sugar impact. The trade-off is often an aftertaste. Best if not heavily relied upon. We'll discuss how to combine them cleverly for optimal taste.

3. **Sugar Alcohols:** Xylitol, erythritol, sorbitol. Not calorie-free, but much slower to digest than sugar. *Important:* Large quantities can have a laxative effect, so moderation is key.

4. **Stevia:** Extracted from a plant, it's incredibly sweet yet virtually blood sugar neutral. Pure forms work best (many blends contain fillers). Can have a subtle bitter aftertaste in excess.

Focus on Fiber: Your Blood Sugar Superpower

Fiber does some heavy lifting for diabetics! Here's the breakdown:

1. **The Slowdown:** Fiber bulks up food and slows its passage through your system, preventing those wild blood sugar spikes.

2. **Heart Health Bonus:** Soluble fiber is amazing for managing cholesterol, a huge concern with diabetes.

3. **The Satiety Factor:** Fiber keeps you full longer, great for banishing cravings that sabotage good habits.

4. **Sources:** We'll cover tons in recipes: Beans, berries, leafy greens, seeds, whole grains…the tastiest stuff!

The Mighty Fats: Snacking Satisfaction

Fat got a bad rap for a long time, but now it's our ally! The *right* fats help:

1. **Energy Sustainer:** Fats slow digestion, making snacks more sustaining, so no hungry meltdown by 11 am!

2. **Blood Sugar Buddy:** Fats actually help moderate how carbs are processed, preventing rollercoaster dips and surges.

3. **Deliciousness Factor:** We're talking avocados, nuts, olive oil…think richness and crave-worthy textures, NOT empty calories.

Beyond "Whole Wheat": Flour Power

Whole wheat was a revolution, but now there's MORE! Let's unlock the secrets of:

1. **Almond Flour:** Perfect for baked treats, low in carbs, full of flavor. It's denser than wheat, so recipes need adapting.

2. **Coconut Flour:** Naturally sweet, super high in fiber. Ultra-absorbent, making recipes extra thirsty!

3. **Oat Flour:** Simple – just grind oats in a blender. Adds hearty texture and mild sweetness.

4. **Other Star Players:** Chickpea flour, buckwheat …a world to explore!

Notes:

- **No Fear:** I want to dispel the myth that a diabetes diagnosis means saying goodbye to enjoyable foods.

- **Empowerment:** Understanding *why* these swaps work builds confidence to modify other favorite recipes.

- **Recipes Ahead!** In the upcoming chapters, we'll put this knowledge into action, showing how to use these powerful ingredients to craft snacks and desserts that nourish both body and soul.

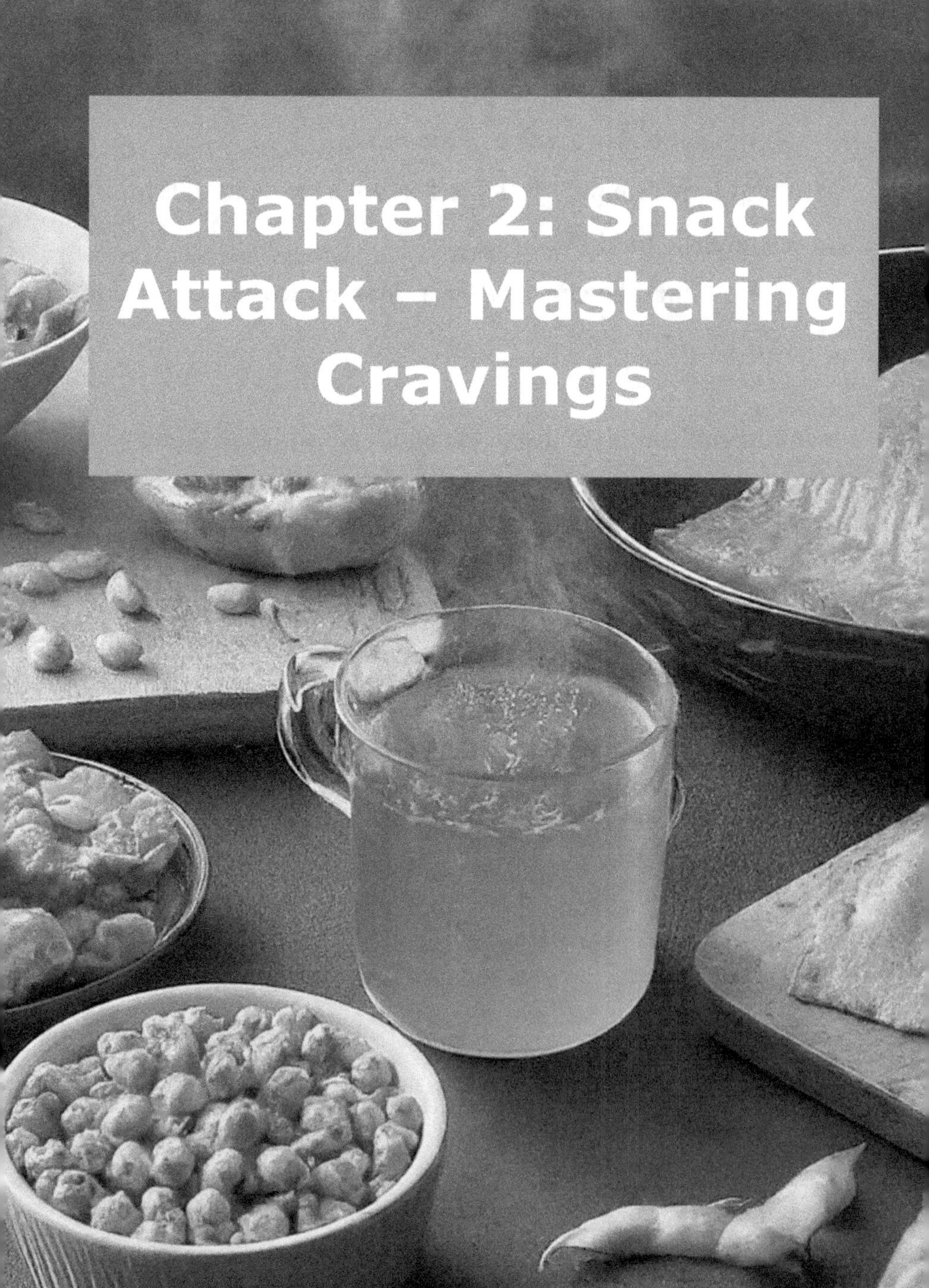

Chapter 2: Snack Attack – Mastering Cravings

Edamame Power Pods

Ingredients:

- 1 cup frozen edamame in the pod
- 1/2 teaspoon of any salt-free seasoning blend (options below)

Spice Option 1: Garlic-Herb

- 1/4 teaspoon dried garlic powder
- 1/4 teaspoon dried oregano or Italian seasoning

Spice Option 2: Fiery Chili

- 1/4 teaspoon chili powder
- 1/8 teaspoon ground cumin
- Pinch of cayenne pepper

Instructions:

1. **Steam & Spice:** Steam the edamame according to package directions. Drain well. While still warm, toss with your chosen seasoning blend.
2. **Enjoy!** Perfect for an on-the-go snack. Pop individual pods from the shell and enjoy the protein-packed beans.

Nutrition (approx. per serving): 120 calories, 5g fat, 11g carbohydrates (8g fiber!), 11g protein. Excellent source of fiber, protein, and iron.

Tips:

- Pre-portion into little baggies for healthy snacking anywhere!
- Fresh edamame pods can also be used when in season.

Prep Time: 10 minutes

Lemony White Bean Dip

Ingredients:

- 1 (15oz) can cannellini beans (white kidney beans) – drained, rinsed
- 1 tablespoon extra virgin olive oil
- 2 tablespoons lemon juice
- 1 clove garlic, minced
- 1 sprig fresh rosemary
- 1 tablespoon tahini (optional)
- Salt and pepper to taste
- Veggies of choice for dipping: carrots, celery, cucumber, whole-wheat pita wedges

Instructions

1. **Blend:** Combine beans, olive oil, lemon juice, garlic, rosemary sprig, and tahini (if using) in a food processor or blender. Process until smooth.
2. **Season:** Taste and adjust salt and pepper as needed. Remove rosemary sprig.
3. **Chill & Serve:** Refrigerate for at least 30 minutes to allow flavors to meld. Serve chilled with your choice of dippers.

Nutrition (approx. per 2 tbsp serving): 100 calories, 6g fat, 10g carbohydrates (4g fiber!), 4g protein. A satisfying way to increase fiber and healthy fats.

Tips:

- For extra brightness, add a sprinkle of lemon zest when serving.

- Omit tahini if desired – adds creaminess but is still yummy without!

Prep Time: 15 minutes (plus chilling)

Tuna Salad Reinvented

Ingredients:

- 1 (5oz) can of tuna, packed in water (drained)
- 1/4 cup plain Greek yogurt
- 2 tablespoons diced celery
- 1 tablespoon diced red onion
- Salt and pepper to taste
- Lettuce cups or cucumber slices for serving

Instructions

1. **Mash & Mix:** In a bowl, mash tuna with a fork. Add Greek yogurt, celery, onion, salt, and pepper. Mix until well combined.
2. **Serve:** Use as a filling for lettuce cups or cucumber slices, creating a refreshing and satisfying lunch or snack.

Nutrition (approx. per 1/2 cup serving): 140 calories, 2.5g fat, 3g carbohydrates (minimal fiber), 24g protein. Excellent source of lean protein.

Tips:

- Add a squeeze of lemon for extra zing.
- Chopped dill or parsley add a delicious fresh herb element.

Prep Time: 10 minutes

Crunchy Chickpea Bites

Ingredients:

- 1 (15oz) can chickpeas, drained and rinsed
- 1 tablespoon extra virgin olive oil
- 1 teaspoon ground cumin
- 1/2 teaspoon smoked paprika
- Pinch of cayenne pepper (optional)
- Salt to taste

Instructions:

1. **Prep & Dry:** Preheat oven to 400°F (200°C). Pat chickpeas dry with a paper towel (this is key for crispiness!)
2. **Toss & Spice:** Toss chickpeas with olive oil, cumin, paprika, cayenne (if using), and a pinch of salt. Spread in a single layer on a baking sheet.
3. **Roast:** Bake for 25-30 minutes, stirring halfway through, until golden brown and crisp.
4. **Cool & Enjoy:** Let cool slightly before enjoying. Perfect for portable snacking!

Nutrition (approx. per 1/4 cup serving): 120 calories, 6g fat, 15g carbohydrates (6g fiber!), 6g protein. Roasting creates crave-worthy texture while providing fiber and some plant-based protein.

Tips:

- Season to taste – play with other spice mixes you love!
- For even more crunch, remove the skins of the chickpeas before roasting (slightly time-consuming but worthwhile if you love extra crispy munchies!)

Prep Time: 15 minutes (plus baking)

Smoked Salmon Roll-Ups

Ingredients:

- 4 ounces smoked salmon, thinly sliced
- 2 ounces low-fat cream cheese, softened
- 1/2 avocado, sliced into thin strips
- 1/4 cup thinly sliced red onion
- Fresh dill or chives (optional)

Instructions:

1. **Spread & Stack:** Spread a thin layer of cream cheese onto each salmon slice. Layer on avocado strips and a sprinkling of red onion.

2. **Roll & Chill:** Carefully roll up and transfer to a plate. Cover and refrigerate for at least 30 minutes to firm up slightly.

3. **Slice & Serve:** Before serving, slice each roll-up into bite-sized pieces. Garnish with fresh herbs for a touch of color.

Nutrition (approx. per 2 roll-ups): 180 calories, 14g fat, 3g carbohydrates (1g fiber!), 11g protein. Good source of healthy omega-3 fats and protein for sustained energy.

Tips:

- Substitute Greek yogurt for cream cheese for a tangier alternative.
- No smoked salmon? Substitute cooked shrimp or even leftover shredded chicken.

Prep Time: 20 minutes (plus chilling)

Blackberry-Chia Parfait

Ingredients:

- 1 cup plain, sugar-free Greek yogurt
- 1/2 cup fresh blackberries (or frozen, thawed)
- 2 tablespoons chia seeds
- Optional toppings: drizzle of honey, chopped nuts, a sprinkle of cinnamon

Instructions:

1. **Layer & Chill:** In a jar or glass, layer yogurt, blackberries, and chia seeds. Repeat for one more layer. Cover and refrigerate for at least 4 hours, or ideally overnight.

2. **Toppings:** Just before serving, add optional toppings such as a drizzle of honey (remember, use honey sparingly if managing diabetes!), a few chopped nuts for crunch, or a touch of cinnamon.

Nutrition (approx. per serving): 200 calories, 8g fat, 20g carbohydrates (10g fiber!), 18g protein. Excellent source of fiber, protein, and those heart-healthy omega-3 fats from the chia seeds.

Tips:

- Swap other berries: Raspberries, blueberries… whatever you love!
- Pre-portion: Prep them in advance for healthy grab-and-go breakfasts or snacks.

Prep Time: 10 minutes (plus chilling time)

Fruit Salsa & Cinnamon Chips

Ingredients:

- 1 cup mixed fruit (diced apples, strawberries, peach chunks)
- 1 tablespoon lime juice
- 1 teaspoon chopped fresh mint
- 4 whole-wheat tortillas
- 1/2 teaspoon cinnamon
- Pinch of stevia or xylitol (optional, for extra sweetness)

Instructions:

1. **Make the Salsa:** Combine chopped fruit, lime juice, and mint in a bowl. Gently toss to mix.

2. **Chips:** Cut tortillas into triangles. Bake in a preheated 350°F (175°C) oven for 8-10 minutes, until crisp. Brush lightly with olive oil if desired, then dust with cinnamon (and the tiniest bit of sweetener if you want a touch more sweetness).

Nutrition (approx. per serving - 1/4 salsa + 2 chips): 160 calories, 2g fat, 32g carbohydrates (6g fiber!), 4g protein. A lighter take on chips and dip, offering antioxidants and fiber!

Tips:

- Any combo of fruit works! Get creative with berries, mango, etc.
- Bake more chips than you need – they make a tasty snack on their own.

Prep Time: 15 minutes (plus baking)

Berry Swirl Smoothies

Ingredients:

- 1 cup frozen mixed berries
- 1 scoop vanilla protein powder (unsweetened or plant-based)
- 1/2 cup unsweetened almond milk (or your choice of milk)
- 1 handful fresh kale
- Optional: drizzle of honey or 1/2 frozen banana for added sweetness

Instructions:

1. **Blend!** Combine all ingredients in a blender and blend until smooth and creamy. If too thick, add a splash of water to thin it out.

Nutrition (approx. per serving): 250 calories, 5g fat, 22g carbohydrates (8g fiber!), 25g protein. A balanced smoothie to refuel after a workout or as a substantial snack.

Tips:

- Make-ahead packs: Pre-portion servings of fruit and kale. Freeze and toss into the blender with the rest for an instant smoothie!
- Swap greens: Any tender leafy green works – spinach, Swiss chard, etc.

Prep Time: 5 minutes

Gingered Pear Bites

Ingredients:

- 2 ripe pears (Anjou or Bartlett variety recommended)
- 1 tablespoon pure maple syrup
- 1/2 teaspoon grated fresh ginger
- Pinch of ground cinnamon
- Plain Greek yogurt for topping (optional)

Instructions:

1. Prep & Bake: Preheat oven to 375°F (190°C). Wash and slice pears in half, core them, and place cut-side-up in a baking dish. Stir maple syrup with ginger and drizzle over pears. Sprinkle with cinnamon. Bake for 20-25 minutes, until softened.

2. Serve Warm: Top with a dollop of plain unsweetened yogurt and enjoy.

Nutrition (approx. per 1/2 pear): 100 calories, 0g fat, 26g carbohydrates (5g fiber!), 1g protein. Naturally sweet, with a spicy twist from the ginger!

Tips:

- Fruit Swap: This method works beautifully with firm apples too.
- Store leftovers in the fridge – enjoy cold with yogurt for breakfast!

Prep Time: 15 minutes (plus baking)

Citrus Burst

Ingredients:

- 1 grapefruit, sectioned
- 1 orange, peeled and sliced
- 1/2 cup unsweetened coconut yogurt
- Optional toppings: chopped pistachios, a sprinkle of unsweetened coconut **flakes**

Instructions:

1. Assemble: Arrange grapefruit and orange in a bowl or plate. Add a generous dollop of unsweetened coconut yogurt (add additional dollops if portioning individual servings).
2. Garnish & Serve: Scatter over your toppings of choice (if using) and serve immediately.

Nutrition (approx. per serving): 160 calories, 8g fat, 23g carbohydrates (5g fiber!), 3g protein. Refreshingly light and packed full of vitamin C!

Tips:

- Other citrus works well: Add tangerine sections, tangelo... whatever looks vibrant at the market.
- Dairy-free? Unsweetened almond or soy yogurt makes a fine substitute.

Prep Time: 10 minutes

Savory-Sweet Trail Mix

Ingredients:

- 1/2 cup roasted almonds (unsalted)
- 1/4 cup pistachios (unsalted, shelled)
- 1/4 cup pepitas (shelled pumpkin seeds)
- 2 tablespoons dried cranberries (unsweetened, or choose unsweetened cherries for a tart option)
- 1 teaspoon Everything Bagel seasoning (choose a no-salt variety if possible)

Instructions:

1. **Combine & Enjoy:** Simply toss all ingredients together in a bowl. Divide into small containers or baggies for convenient, on-the-go snacking.

Nutrition (approx. per 1/4 cup serving): 180 calories, 14g fat, 13g carbohydrates (3g fiber!), 8g protein. A satisfying mix of fats, protein, and a hint of sweetness for sustained energy.

Tips:

- Get creative with nuts and seeds: Substitute cashews, pecans, etc., based on your preference.
- Sweetness Control: Increase or decrease dried fruit based on your preference. If using sweetened cranberries, use a very small amount and balance with more seeds/nuts.

Prep Time: 5 minutes

Tropical Energy Bites

Ingredients:

- 1/2 cup unsweetened dried pineapple, finely chopped
- 1/4 cup unsweetened coconut flakes
- 1/4 cup shredded almonds
- 1 tablespoon fresh lime juice
- Additional coconut flakes for rolling (optional)

Instructions:

1. **Mix & Form:** Combine all ingredients (except additional coconut flakes) in a bowl until a slightly sticky dough forms. Shape into bite-sized balls.

2. **Optional Roll:** For extra coconut goodness, roll your bites in a plate of unsweetened coconut flakes.

Nutrition (approx. per ball): 80 calories, 6g fat, 7g carbohydrates (2g fiber!), 2g protein. A portable dose of tropical flavor and healthy fats to keep you going.

Tips:

- Sweetness Boost:** A tiny addition of chopped dates would amplify the natural sweetness, adjust for blood sugar if using!
- Make-Ahead: Store in the fridge for up to a week for grab-and-go satisfaction.

Prep Time: 15 minutes

Cocoa Roast Almonds

Ingredients:

- 1 cup raw almonds
- 1 tablespoon unsweetened cocoa powder
- Pinch of stevia or xylitol (to taste)
- 1/4 teaspoon ground cinnamon

Instructions:

1. **Flavor Boost:** In a bowl, toss almonds with cocoa powder, sweetener, and cinnamon, coating evenly. Spread in a single layer on a baking sheet.
2. **Roast:** Bake in a preheated 350°F (175°C) oven for 10-12 minutes, stirring halfway through, until fragrant and slightly darkened. Let cool completely before storing in an airtight container.

Nutrition (approx. per 1/4 cup serving): 180 calories, 15g fat, 10g carbohydrates (4g fiber!), 8g protein. Chocolatey flavor with just a hint of sweetness.

Tips:

- Spice It Up: A pinch of chili powder adds a delightful kick!
- Use your choice of nut: This method works with pecans, walnuts, or cashews.

Prep Time: 5 minutes (plus baking/roasting)

Spiced Walnuts

Ingredients:

- 1 cup walnut halves
- 1 tablespoon olive oil
- 1/2 teaspoon smoked paprika
- 1/4 teaspoon erythritol (or alternative sweetener to taste)
- Pinch of salt (optional)

Instructions:

1. **Flavor Coat:** Toss walnuts with olive oil, paprika, sweetener, and a pinch of salt (if using) in a bowl, making sure they're evenly coated.

2. **Roast & Toast:** Spread nuts in a single layer on a baking sheet. Bake in a preheated oven at 325°F (160°C) for 12-15 minutes, stirring once, until walnuts are fragrant and lightly toasted. Let cool completely before storing in an airtight container.

Nutrition (approx. per 1/4 cup serving): 190 calories, 18g fat, 4g carbohydrates (2g fiber!), 4g protein. An addictive crunchy snack and fantastic salad or yogurt topping.

Tips:

- Spice Swaps: Play with warm spices like cumin, coriander, or a touch of ground cardamom.
- Savory Option: Omit the sweetener for a strictly savory flavor profile; great on salad!

Prep Time: 5 minutes (plus baking and cooling)

Sunflower Seed Power

Ingredients:

- 1 cup raw, shelled sunflower seeds
- 1 teaspoon your favorite salt-free herb blend (Italian, lemon-pepper, etc.)

Instructions:

1. **Toast & Toss:** Heat a dry skillet over medium heat. Add sunflower seeds and toast for 2-3 minutes, stirring constantly, until lightly golden and fragrant. Immediately remove from heat and toss with your preferred herb blend.

2. **Cool & Enjoy:** Spread to cool completely on a sheet of parchment paper and enjoy once fully cooled. Store leftovers in an airtight container.

Nutrition (approx. per 1/4 cup serving): 160 calories, 14g fat, 6g carbohydrates (3g fiber!), 6g protein. A satisfying burst of healthy fats and great source of vitamins and minerals.

Tips:

- WATCH THOSE SEEDS! They go from golden to burned in a flash, keep a close eye and stir.
- Experiment: Make mini batches with different herb blends to find your favorite flavor combos.

Prep Time: 10 minutes

- **Blood Sugar Friendly:** Focus on healthy fats, protein, and fiber to slow digestion and avoid rapid spikes.

- **Portion Control:** Easy to make in advance and divide for balanced snacking.

- **Variety is Key:** Prevents boredom and allows for tailored nutrient delivery.

Avocado Ranch

Ingredients

- 1 ripe avocado, halved and pitted
- 1 packet sugar-free ranch dressing mix
- 1/4 cup plain Greek yogurt
- 1 tablespoon lemon juice
- Salt and pepper to taste

Instructions:

1. **Mash & Mix:** Scoop avocado flesh into a bowl and mash until smooth. Add ranch dressing mix, Greek yogurt, lemon juice, and season with a pinch of salt and pepper. Stir until well combined.

2. **Adjust & Serve:** Taste and add more lemon juice or seasoning if desired. For a thinner consistency, stir in a bit of water. Enjoy immediately, or chill for later use.

Nutrition (approx. per 2 tbsp serving): 80 calories, 7g fat, 4g carbohydrates (2g fiber!), 2g protein. All the creamy, tangy ranch flavor at a fraction of the calories found in traditional versions.

Tips:

- Garnish: Sprinkling chopped fresh herbs adds a gourmet touch.
- Veggie Dip: This makes an excellent vegetable dip. Serve with crudités for a satisfying snack.

Prep Time: 10 minutes

Baba Ganoush Twist

Ingredients:

- 1 medium eggplant
- 2 tablespoons tahini
- 1 clove garlic, minced
- 2 tablespoons lemon juice
- 1/2 teaspoon ground cumin
- Salt and pepper to taste

Instructions:

1. **Roast & Scoop:** Pierce eggplant with a fork and roast whole in a preheated 400°F (200°C) oven for 40-50 minutes, until tender. Slice in half lengthwise and scoop out the flesh.

2. **Blend & Season:** In a food processor or blender, combine roasted eggplant flesh, tahini, garlic, lemon juice, cumin, salt, and pepper. Blend until smooth and creamy.

Nutrition (approx. per 1/4 cup serving): 80 calories, 6g fat, 7g carbohydrates (3g fiber!), 2g protein. The satisfying smokiness of the original, without all the added oil.

Tips:

- Serving Suggestion: Drizzle with extra olive oil and a sprinkle of toasted sesame seeds for added dimension. Delicious with whole-wheat pita bread or veggie sticks.

- Storage: Baba ganoush keeps well in the fridge for a few days.

Prep Time: 15 minutes (plus roasting)

Spicy Beet Hummus

Ingredients:

- 1 medium beet, roasted (or use pre-cooked, packaged beets)
- 1 (15oz) can chickpeas, drained and rinsed
- 1/4 cup olive oil
- 2 tablespoons lemon juice
- 1 clove garlic, minced
- 1/4 teaspoon ground cumin (optional)
- Pinch of cayenne pepper, or more to taste
- Salt and pepper to taste

Instructions:

1. **Process & Spice:** Roughly chop the roasted beet. Add it to a food processor or blender, along with the remaining ingredients. Process until smooth. Adjust salt, pepper, and cayenne to your preferred heat level.

2. **Garnish & Serve:** Transfer to a serving bowl and drizzle with olive oil. Sprinkle with a pinch of paprika for color. Excellent dip for tortilla chips, crackers, or veggies.

Nutrition (approx. per 1/4 cup serving): 140 calories, 9g fat, 15g carbohydrates (5g fiber!), 3g protein. Vibrant color, earthy flavor, and a boost of fiber!

Tips

- No Roasting? Pre-cooked, packaged beets work too!
- Swap Lemon for Lime: Substitute lime juice for a fresh, tangy variation.

Prep Time: 15 minutes (if using pre-cooked beets)

Recipe 4: Protein Ranch Crackers

Ingredients:

- 1 cup almond flour
- 1/4 cup protein powder (vanilla or unflavored works best)
- 1 tablespoon dried herbs (choose Italian, ranch, or your favorite combo)
- 1 tablespoon olive oil
- 2-3 tablespoons water
- Pinch of salt

Instructions:

1. **Make the Dough:** Combine almond flour, protein powder, herbs, olive oil, and salt in a bowl. Gradually add water, 1 tablespoon at a time, and knead until the dough comes together. Don't overmix; it should be smooth but not sticky.

2. **Roll & Cut:** Roll the dough between two sheets of parchment paper (lightly floured) until very thin, about 1/8 inch. Using a knife or pizza cutter, cut into squares or desired shapes.

3. **Bake:** Transfer crackers to a baking sheet lined with parchment. Bake in a preheated oven at 350°F (175°C) for 12-15 minutes, or until crispy and lightly browned.

Nutrition (approx. per 4 crackers): 110 calories, 7g fat, 7g carbohydrates (2g fiber!), 6g protein. Crispy, satisfying vehicles to enhance your favorite dips, adding a little boost of protein to the snack spread.

Tips:

- Flavor Them Up: Experiment with spices – garlic powder, onion powder, etc.
- Storage: Store crackers in an airtight container at room temperature for several days.

Prep Time: 20 minutes (plus baking)

Roasted Pepper Spread

Ingredients:

- 2 large red bell peppers
- 1/4 cup plain Greek yogurt
- 1 clove garlic, roasted (or use jarred roasted garlic)
- 1 teaspoon balsamic vinegar
- Salt and pepper to taste

Instructions:

1. **Char & Peel:** Roast red peppers over an open flame (stovetop works!), under a broiler, or in a hot oven (450°F/230°C) until skins are charred and blistered. Place in a bowl, cover tightly, and let steam for 10 minutes. Once cool, peel and remove seeds and stems.

2. **Blend & Flavor:** In a food processor or blender, combine roasted peppers, yogurt, roasted garlic, vinegar, salt, and pepper. Blend until smooth and creamy. Taste and adjust seasonings.

Nutrition (approx. per 1/4 cup serving): 35 calories, 1g fat, 6g carbohydrates (2g fiber!), 2g protein. A lighter, tangy alternative to creamy dips. Great with whole-grain crackers or crisp vegetables.

Tips:

- Make-Ahead: This spread tastes even better after marinating in the fridge for a few hours.

- Mix-In Variety: For extra depth, add a handful of fresh herbs like basil or parsley.

Prep Time: 15 minutes (plus pepper roasting)

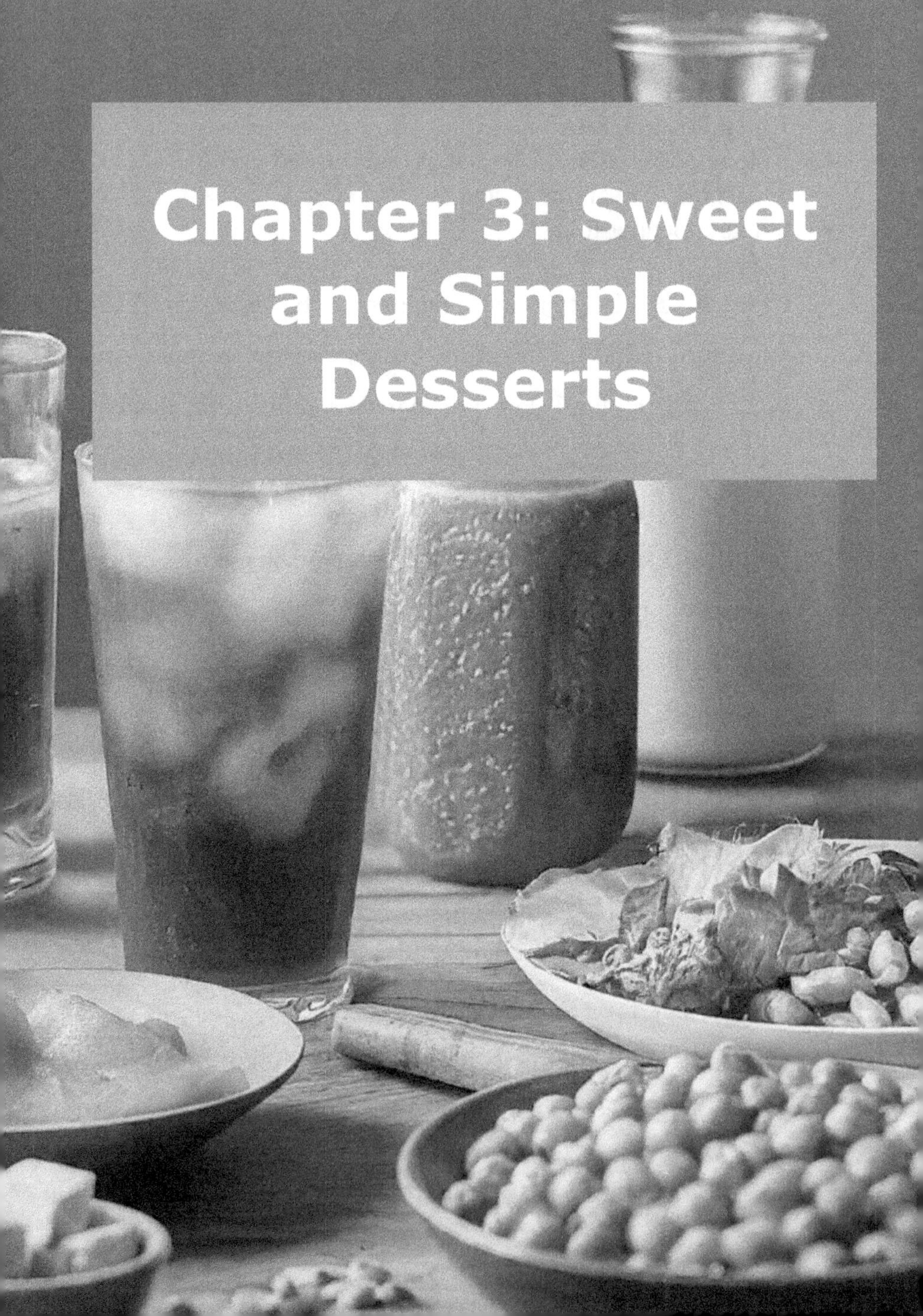

Chapter 3: Sweet and Simple Desserts

Recipe 1: Oatmeal Raisin Reimagined

Ingredients:

- 1 cup rolled oats (or use quick oats)
- 1/2 cup unsweetened applesauce or mashed ripe banana
- 1/4 cup raisins
- 1 tablespoon pure maple syrup
- 1 teaspoon ground cinnamon
- 1/2 teaspoon vanilla extract
- Pinch of salt
- Optional add-ins: chopped walnuts, a sprinkle of ground flaxseed

Instructions:

1. **Mix & Bake:** Combine all ingredients in a bowl. For individual portions, divide the batter into muffin cups, ramekins, or small baking dishes. Bake in a preheated oven at 350°F (175°C) for 20-25 minutes, or until golden and set.
2. **Make Ahead:** For hot oatmeal on the go, make a big batch, portion into small containers, and refrigerate. Reheat with a splash of milk, add toppings, and enjoy.

Nutrition (approx. per serving - muffin-size): 180 calories, 6g fat, 32g carbohydrates (4g fiber!), 4g protein. A warm, wholesome breakfast with the classic raisin sweetness.

Tips:

- No Raisins? Substitute dried cranberries, chopped dates, or diced plums.

- Use Ground Oats: Grind in a blender or food processor for a porridge-like texture.

Prep Time: 10 minutes (plus baking)

Recipe 2: Carrot Cake Protein Muffins

Ingredients:

- 1 cup grated carrots
- 1/2 cup unsweetened applesauce
- 1/2 cup coconut flour
- 1/4 cup protein powder (vanilla or unflavored)
- 2 eggs
- 1 teaspoon cinnamon
- 1/2 teaspoon nutmeg
- 1/4 teaspoon ground ginger
- 1/4 teaspoon baking powder
- Pinch of salt
- Stevia or monk fruit sweetener to taste

Instructions:

1. **Batter Up:** In a bowl, combine all ingredients until a batter forms. Sweetener adjustments should be based on preferred level of sweetness.

2. **Fill & Bake:** Grease a muffin tin, then scoop batter into each cup, filling about 2/3 way. Bake in a preheated 350°F (175°C) oven for 20-25 minutes, until golden and a toothpick inserted in the center comes out clean.

Nutrition (approx. per muffin): 120 calories, 5g fat, 10g carbohydrates (2g fiber!), 8g protein. Sneak in extra veggies while hitting those protein goals with this satisfying morning treat.

Tips:

- Spice Swap: Use your favorite pumpkin pie spice blend instead of individual spices.

- Frosting Upgrade: Whisk cream cheese with Greek yogurt and a hint of sweetener for a healthy topping.

Prep Time: 15 minutes (plus baking)

Recipe 3: Blueberry Lemon Bars

Ingredients (Crust):

- 1 cup almond flour
- 1/4 cup unsweetened shredded coconut
- 2 tablespoons coconut oil, melted
- 1 teaspoon lemon extract

Ingredients (Filling):

- 1 cup fresh or frozen blueberries
- 2 eggs
- 1 tablespoon lemon zest
- 2 tablespoons honey or maple syrup
- Optional: 1 teaspoon arrowroot powder (thickens if blueberries are very juicy)

Instructions:

1. **Make the Crust:** Combine crust ingredients, press into a greased 8x8 baking dish lined with parchment. Bake at 350°F(175°C) for 10-12 minutes, just until edges are golden.

2. **Prepare Filling:** Whisk together filling ingredients in a bowl. Gently fold in blueberries. Pour filling over partially baked crust, spread evenly. Bake for an additional 20-25 minutes, or until filling is set and lightly browned. Let cool completely before slicing.

Nutrition (approx. per bar): 130 calories, 9g fat, 12g carbohydrates (2g fiber!), 2g protein. Tart, fruity perfection on a satisfying, grain-free crust.

Tips

- Sweet Swaps: Adjust sweetener level to your liking, substitute other berries if desired.
- Serve-Cold:** These bars taste best chilled! Store in the fridge and enjoy them cold.

Prep Time: 15 minutes (plus baking/cooling)

Recipe 4: Peanut Butter Chocolate Chip Cookies

Ingredients:

- 1 ripe banana, mashed
- 1/2 cup unsweetened peanut butter (creamy or crunchy!)
- 1 egg
- 1/2 cup rolled oats
- 1/4 cup dark chocolate chips (at least 70% cacao)
- 1/4 teaspoon vanilla extract
- Pinch of salt
- Xylitol or stevia to taste (start with a small amount)

Instructions:

1. Mix, Scoop, Bake: In a bowl, combine all ingredients until a dough forms. If too wet, add a bit more oats, if too dry, a splash of milk of choice. Roll into balls, slightly flatten onto a baking sheet, and bake in a preheated 350°F (175°C) oven for 12-15 minutes, or until lightly golden. Cool slightly before enjoying.

Nutrition (approx. per cookie): 100 calories, 6g fat, 10g carbohydrates (2g fiber!), 3g protein. Simple, peanut buttery goodness to satisfy those occasional cookie cravings.

Tips:

- Other Nut Butters: Almond butter, cashew butter - play around!
- Sweetness is Personal: This recipe is a starting point, adjust sweetener based on taste.

Prep Time: 10 minutes (plus baking)

Recipe 5: Apple Crumble Revisited

Ingredients (Filling):

- 2 cups apples, peeled and diced
- 1 tablespoon lemon juice
- 1 tablespoon pure maple syrup
- 1 teaspoon cinnamon
- Pinch of salt

Ingredients (Crumble):

- 1/2 cup oats (rolled or quick oats)
- 1/4 cup almond flour
- 1 tablespoon cinnamon
- 2 tablespoons chopped nuts (optional)
- 2 tablespoons cold, unsalted butter (cubed) or coconut oil

Instructions:

1. Toss the Fruit: Combine filling ingredients in a small baking dish.

2. Create Crumble: Combine oats, almond flour, cinnamon, and nuts in a bowl. With a pastry cutter or your fingers, blend in the cubed butter (or coconut oil) until it resembles coarse crumbs.

3. Bake & Serve: Scatter crumble over apples. Bake in a preheated 375°F (190°C) oven for 25-30 minutes, or until fruit is tender and topping is golden brown. For a little extra

decadence, serve warm with a scoop of light vanilla ice cream or a dollop of plain yogurt.

Nutrition (approx. per serving without ice cream): 200 calories, 10g fat, 26g carbohydrates (5g fiber!), 3g protein. Cozy, comforting flavors with a lightened-up sweetness.

Tips:

- Variety is Key: Different apples (tart Granny Smith, sweet Honeycrisp, etc.) change the flavor profile.
- Pre-Portion: Bake crumbles in individual ramekins for portion control.

Prep Time: 15 minutes (plus baking)

Recipe 1: Avocado Chocolate Mousse

Ingredients:

- 1 ripe avocado, halved and pitted
- 1/4 cup unsweetened cocoa powder
- 2 tablespoons pure maple syrup (or sweetener of choice)
- 1 tablespoon unsweetened almond milk (or milk of choice)
- 1/2 teaspoon vanilla extract
- Pinch of salt

Instructions:

1. **Blend for Bliss:** Scoop avocado flesh into a blender or food processor. Add cocoa powder, sweetener, milk, vanilla extract, and salt. Blend until incredibly smooth and creamy. Taste and adjust sweetener if needed.

2. **Chill Out:** Refrigerate for at least 30 minutes to thicken and enhance those chocolate flavors.

Nutrition (approx. per serving - divides into 2): 150 calories, 12g fat, 16g carbohydrates (7g fiber!), 3g protein. Decadent yet surprisingly nutritious!

Tips:

- Toppings Galore: Dollop of coconut whipped cream, chopped nuts, a sprinkle of cinnamon...get creative!

- Avocado Matters: Choose a perfectly ripe avocado – creamy, not watery or with browning.

Prep Time: 10 minutes (plus chilling)

Recipe 2: Black Bean Brownies

Ingredients:

- 1 (15oz) can black beans, drained and rinsed
- 2 eggs
- 1/4 cup unsweetened cocoa powder
- 1/4 cup pure maple syrup
- 1 teaspoon vanilla extract
- 1/4 teaspoon baking powder
- Pinch of salt
- Optional: 1/4 cup dark chocolate chips

Instructions:

1. **Secret Ingredient:** Preheat oven to 350°F (175°C). Grease an 8x8 baking pan. In a blender or food processor, purée black beans until smooth. Stir in eggs, cocoa powder, maple syrup, vanilla, baking powder, and salt until well combined. Fold in the chocolate chips (if using).

2. **Bake & Devour:** Pour batter into the prepared pan and bake for 25-30 minutes, or until a toothpick inserted in the center comes out with just a few moist crumbs. Let cool completely before slicing – they'll firm up perfectly!

Nutrition (approx. per brownie): 120 calories, 4g fat, 18g carbohydrates (5g fiber!), 5g protein. Don't knock it till you try it! Incredibly dense, fudgy, and no bean flavor whatsoever.

Tips:

- Sweetness Level: Start with minimal sweetness and adjust the next time depending on your preference.

- Frosting Hack: Whip Greek yogurt with cocoa powder and sweetener for a healthy topping.

Prep Time: 15 minutes (plus baking/cooling)

Recipe 3: Cocoa Energy Bites

Ingredients:

- 1 cup rolled oats
- 1/2 cup nut butter (peanut, almond, or your favorite)
- 1/4 cup dark chocolate chips
- 2 tablespoons unsweetened cocoa powder
- 2 tablespoons agave or maple syrup
- 1 teaspoon vanilla extract

Instructions:

1. **Combine & Form:** Combine all ingredients in a bowl and mix thoroughly until a slightly sticky dough forms. Roll the dough into bite-sized balls (about 1 tablespoon each).
2. **Chill & Store:** Place on a baking sheet lined with parchment and refrigerate to firm up (about 30 minutes). Store in an airtight container in the refrigerator.

Nutrition (approx. per ball): 100 calories, 6g fat, 12g carbohydrates (2g fiber!), 3g protein. Portable little bursts of chocolatey goodness and sustained energy.

Tips:

- Mix-In Madness: Add shredded coconut, chopped dried fruit, mini pretzels... the possibilities are endless!
- Make-Ahead: These keep well in the fridge for a week, perfect for pre-workout snacks.

Recipe 4: Hot Cocoa Reimagined

Ingredients:

- 1 cup unsweetened almond milk (or milk of your choice)
- 2 tablespoons unsweetened cocoa powder
- 1 teaspoon pure maple syrup (or your preferred sweetener)
- 1/4 teaspoon vanilla extract
- Optional: Pinch of peppermint extract

Instructions

1. Flavor Magic: Combine all ingredients in a small saucepan over medium heat. Whisk gently until everything is dissolved and heated through. Taste and adjust for sweetness if needed.

2. Get Frothy: For an extra creamy texture, blitz with an immersion blender or give it a whirl in a regular blender before serving.

Nutrition (approx. per serving): 80 calories, 2g fat, 14g carbohydrates (1g fiber!), 3g protein. Way more satisfying than those sugar-laden packets!

Tips:

- Spice it Up: Add a pinch of cinnamon, nutmeg, or any warm spice you love.
- Dairy-Free Swap: Coconut milk is another great option for this recipe.

Prep Time: 5 minutes

Recipe 5: Cacao Nib Trail Mix

Ingredients:

- 1/4 cup dark chocolate chunks (at least 70% cacao)
- 1/4 cup dried berries (cranberries, blueberries, cherries, etc.)
- 1/4 cup raw cacao nibs
- 1/2 cup mixed nuts (almonds, walnuts, pecans, etc.)

Instructions:

1. Combine!: Simply toss all ingredients together in a bowl. Divide into small, portable snack bags or containers.

Nutrition (approx. per 1/4 cup serving): 200 calories, 14g fat, 16g carbohydrates (5g fiber!), 6g protein. Sweet, salty, crunchy, and even a touch bitter (which is surprisingly wonderful with the chocolate!)

Tips:

- Get Creative: Mix up the nuts and fruits, add toasted coconut flakes, or a tiny sprinkle of dried chili flakes for warmth.
- Bulk Up: This scales easily! Make a big batch for easy grab-and-go snacking.

Recipe 1: Strawberry Banana Pops

Ingredients:

- 1 cup strawberries, hulled

- 1 large ripe banana, sliced

- Optional: Splash of milk (dairy or plant-based) for added creaminess

Instructions:

1. **Blend & Freeze:** Blend the strawberries and banana (and milk, if using) in a blender or food processor until completely smooth. Pour the mixture into popsicle molds. Insert popsicle sticks and freeze for at least 4 hours, or until completely solid.

Nutrition (approx. per pop - makes about 4): 80 calories, 0.5g fat, 19g carbohydrates (3g fiber!), 1g protein. Nature's candy in frozen form!

Tips:

- Other Berries Work: Blueberries, raspberries... mix and match to your liking.

- Swirl it Up: Layer different berry purees or a little yogurt for a marbled effect.

Prep Time: 10 minutes (plus freezing)

Recipe 2: Coconut-Lime Sorbet

Ingredients:

- 1 (14oz) can full-fat coconut milk
- 1/4 cup lime juice
- 2 tablespoons lime zest
- 2 tablespoons pure maple syrup (or sweetener of choice)
- Pinch of salt

Instructions (Ice Cream Maker Version):

1. **Chill & Churn:** Chill all ingredients thoroughly. Combine in an ice cream maker and churn according to the manufacturer's instructions. Once thickened, transfer to a freezer-safe container and freeze for at least 2 hours for optimal scooping texture.

Instructions (Granita Version):

1. **Freeze & Scrape:** Combine ingredients in a shallow freezer-safe dish. Freeze for 2 hours, then use a fork to scrape the mixture into icy flakes. Freeze for another hour, then scrape again, creating a fluffy granita consistency.

Nutrition (approx. per 1/2 cup serving): 150 calories, 12g fat, 14g carbohydrates (1g fiber!), 1g protein. A tangy pick-me-up on a hot day.

Tips:

- No Ice Cream Maker? The granita method is delicious & refreshing (though less creamy).
- Garnish Game: Fresh mint leaves add a beautiful touch of color.

Prep Time: 10 minutes (plus freezing)

Recipe 3: "Nice Cream" Base

Ingredients:

- 2 medium ripe bananas, sliced and frozen
- Optional: a splash of your favorite milk (dairy or plant-based) for creaminess

Instructions:

1. **Creamy Churn:** Place frozen bananas (and milk, if using) in a food processor or high-powered blender and blend until smooth and creamy, scraping down the sides as needed. Stop once it resembles the texture of soft-serve ice cream.

Nutrition (approx. per 1/2 cup serving): 110 calories, 1g fat, 26g carbohydrates (4g fiber!), 1g protein. Nature's miraculous dairy-free ice cream alternative!

Endless Mix-in Ideas:

- Chocoholic: Cocoa powder + mini chocolate chips
- Nutty: Peanut butter swirl
- Fruity Burst: Mashed berries of any kind
- Tropical: Mango chunks + a hint of lime juice

Tips:

- Bananas Matter: For the creamiest results, use extra ripe bananas – those brown spots are your friend!
- Blend Then Add: Mix-ins are best stirred in right at the end to prevent getting over blended.

Prep Time: 5 minutes (plus banana freezing)

Recipe 4: Mango-Pineapple Popsicles

Ingredients:

- 1 cup mango chunks (fresh or frozen)
- 1 cup pineapple chunks (fresh or frozen)
- 1 cup plain Greek yogurt

Instructions:

1. For Puree & Swirl: Blend half the mango and half the pineapple separately until each is smooth, then layer those purees with the yogurt, creating swirls in popsicle molds. Insert sticks and freeze as with other pops.

2. For Chunks & Layers: Finely dice the fruit and combine. In popsicle molds, alternate adding a bit of diced fruit with layers of yogurt for a lovely contrasting pattern. Insert the sticks and freeze until solid.

Nutrition (approx. per pop - makes about 4): 120 calories, 2g fat, 22g carbohydrates (3g fiber!), 5g protein. Creamy, tropical deliciousness on a stick!

Tips:

- Fresh vs. Frozen: Both will work, and it can be a combo - fresh with frozen yogurt gives a great texture contrast.
- Sweetness Boost: If fruits aren't super sweet, a drizzle of honey into the puree layers creates extra flavor.

Prep Time: 15 minutes (plus freezing)

Recipe 1: Chia Seed Pudding

Ingredients:

- 1/4 cup chia seeds
- 1 cup unsweetened almond milk (or milk of choice)
- 1/2 cup mashed berries (strawberries, raspberries, blueberries, etc.)
- 1/4 teaspoon ground cinnamon
- Vanilla extract (optional)
- Sweetener of choice to taste (stevia, maple syrup, etc.)

Instructions:

1. **Soak & Swirl:** In a jar or bowl, combine chia seeds with milk, a dash of cinnamon, and a few drops of vanilla (optional). Sweeten to taste, adding very small amounts at first. If desired, gently stir in some mashed berries for a marbled effect.

2. **Chill & Set:** Cover and refrigerate for at least 4 hours, ideally overnight, until pudding thickens. Once it has set, give it a quick stir. Spoon into a glass, and top with remaining mashed berries and sprinkle with cinnamon before serving.

Nutrition (approx. per serving): 180 calories, 10g fat, 20g carbohydrates (11g fiber!), 8g protein. Chia seeds are fiber superstars, making this a breakfast or snack that keeps you feeling full.

Tips:

- Flavor Swaps: Get creative with other spices, cocoa powder, coconut flakes…the options are endless!
- Make-Ahead Meal: Perfect for prepping breakfast the night before for a grab-and-go morning meal.

Prep Time: 10 minutes (plus at least 4 hours for soaking)

Recipe 2: Sugar-Free Fruit Pudding

Ingredients:

- 1 packet sugar-free pudding mix (choose your favorite flavor!)
- 2 cups unsweetened plant-based milk (almond, soy, etc.)
- Optional toppings: fresh fruit, a sprinkle of granola, toasted nuts...

Instructions:

1. **Prepare & Thicken:** Follow the package instructions, substituting unsweetened plant-based milk for regular milk. Refrigerate to allow the pudding to thicken. When serving, add your favorite fruit, a sprinkle of granola, or crushed nuts for texture and crunch.

Nutrition: Varies depending on specific pudding brand and added toppings. Look for puddings low in sugar and higher in protein.

Tips:

- Check the Ingredients: Some "sugar-free" puddings still have refined carbs. Check for whole food sweeteners like stevia and monk fruit if possible.
- Small Portion: These are best enjoyed as occasional treats rather than a regular dietary staple.

Prep Time: 5 minutes (plus setting in the fridge)

Recipe 3: Chocolate Avocado Parfait

Ingredients (Mousse):

- 1 ripe avocado, halved and pitted
- 1/4 cup unsweetened cocoa powder
- 2 tablespoons sweetener of choice (maple syrup, stevia, etc.)
- 1 tablespoon unsweetened plant-based milk
- Pinch of salt
- Ingredients (Parfait):
- Sliced strawberries
- Crushed walnuts

Instructions:

1. **Mousse Magic:** Scoop avocado flesh into a food processor or blender. Add the rest of the mousse ingredients and blend until silky smooth.

2. **Build & Enjoy:** In a glass or bowl, layer the mousse with sliced strawberries and sprinkle with crushed walnuts. Repeat the layers for a visual masterpiece!

Nutrition (approx. per serving): 250 calories, 18g fat, 24g carbohydrates (10g fiber!), 5g protein. Decadent but surprisingly good for you with healthy fats and fiber.

Tips:

- Avocado Matters: Make sure it's perfectly ripe - not too hard, not too mushy.
- Toppings Variety: Other berries, banana slices, whipped coconut cream... endless possibilities!

Prep Time: 15 minutes

Recipe 4: Greek Yogurt Mousse

Ingredients (Mousse):

- 2 cups plain Greek yogurt (low-fat or full-fat)
- 2 tablespoons unsweetened cocoa powder
- 1-2 tablespoons sweetener of choice (honey, maple syrup, stevia, etc.)
- 1/2 teaspoon vanilla extract
- Ingredients (Berry Sauce):
- 1 cup berries of choice (raspberries, blueberries, mixed berries, etc.)
- 1 teaspoon lemon juice
- Sweetener of choice to taste (optional)

Instructions (Mousse):

1. **Sweet & Fluffy:** In a bowl, whisk together Greek yogurt, cocoa powder, sweetener, and vanilla extract until light and fully combined.

Instructions (Berry Sauce):

1. **Simple Berry Blast:** Combine berries and lemon juice in a saucepan and cook over medium-low heat, lightly mashing with a fork. If you want a smoother sauce, blend it briefly. Sweeten to taste (optional depending on fruit).

Assemble & Enjoy: Spoon the mousse into serving glasses or dishes. Top with a generous dollop of berry sauce and serve immediately.

Nutrition (approx. per serving): 190 calories, 6g fat, 20g carbohydrates (2g fiber!), 18g protein. High-protein dessert or snack that feels indulgent!

Tips:

- Citrus Kick: A hint of orange zest in the mousse adds brightness and flavor.
- Sauce It Up: Play with different fruits and adjust the sweetness of the sauce to your preference.

Prep Time: 15 minutes

Recipe 5: PB&J Parfait

Ingredients:

- 1 cup plain Greek yogurt
- 1 tablespoon sugar-free jelly (any flavor you love)
- 1 tablespoon chopped unsalted peanuts

Instructions:

1. **Layer & Swirl:** In a tall glass or dish, layer yogurt with a small amount of the jelly. Swirl gently with a spoon. Repeat until it's nearly full.
2. **Sprinkle & Crunch:** Top with a sprinkle of chopped peanuts and an extra bit of jelly.

Nutrition (approx. per serving): 190 calories, 8g fat, 15g carbohydrates (2g fiber!), 17g protein. All that classic PB & J taste with less sugar.

Tips:

- Nut Swap: Roasted almonds, cashews... whatever you enjoy most!
- Jelly Mix: Mashing fresh berries with a hint of sweetener offers a less processed alternative to some store-bought jellies.

Prep Time: 5 minutes

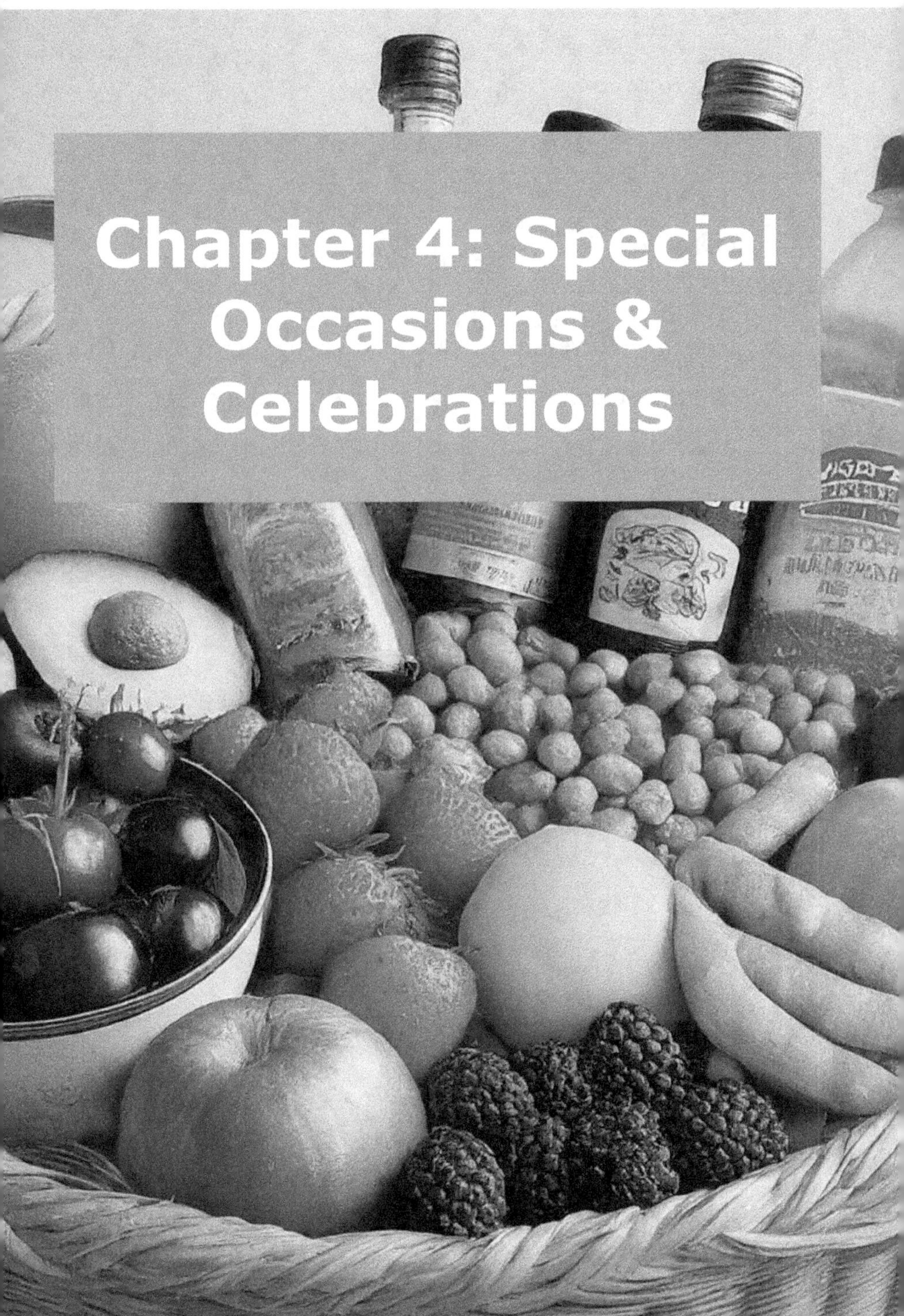
Chapter 4: Special Occasions & Celebrations

♥ **The 'Better' Base:** Instead of heavily processed cake mixes, explore recipes with a foundation of oat flour, almond flour, or whole wheat flour with yogurt or applesauce for moistness.

♥ **Frosting Revamp:** Cream cheese lightened with Greek yogurt, a touch of natural sweeteners, and flavorful extracts make great bases. A tiny bit of real buttercream for rich accents goes a long way.

♥ **Funfetti Upgrade:** Grind unsweetened, freeze-dried strawberries into dust and add to a basic vanilla, yogurt-based frosting! Natural color and tartness balance the sweetness.

♥ **Fruit Takes Center Stage:** Instead of cakes layered with heavy frosting, think a light cake base that allows fresh berries and a dollop of lightly sweetened whipped cream to be the star attraction.

Flavorful Festivities

- ♥ **Theme Treats:** A red velvet cake base using beet for color...pumpkin muffins in fall.... the possibilities are endless, often with surprising natural ingredients that limit added sugar.

- ♥ **Rethink Classics:** "Sugar" cookies in cute holiday shapes using less sweet dough, decorated with yogurt-based glazes colored with fruit/veg concentrates and natural sprinkles.

- ♥ **Portion-Perfect Pies:** Mini muffin-tin pies make individual pumpkin or fruit-based fillings possible, or one full-size pie cut into slivers for everyone to enjoy a taste.

- ♥ **The Spice Factor:** Many holiday flavors rely more on spices (cinnamon, cloves, etc.) than heaps of sugar. Using warm, inviting spices as the focus will make any sweet dish feel more festive.

Mindful Indulgences

- ♥ **The Tasting Plate:** A few squares of chocolate, one small sweet cookie, a spoonful of festive pie...this keeps treats from being off-limits but allows for enjoyment with a focus on the experience, not deprivation.

- ♥ **Savory Balance:** Always provide appealing non-sweet snack options when the focus is sweet treats. Veggie trays, cheese and whole-grain crackers, popcorn...this helps moderate blood sugar.

- ♥ **Mindful Sips:** Festive holiday drinks should have diabetes-friendly options! Sugar-free flavorings in sparkling water, unsweetened festive teas, etc., feel part of the party but won't sabotage blood sugar goals.

Gifts from the Kitchen

1. **Spiced Nuts:** Flavored pecans with sugar-free spice mixes provide a satisfying, low-glycemic treat. Packaging in little jars offers a homemade touch.

2. **DIY Trail Mix:** Bulk purchase of your favorite "safe" nuts, seeds, and dried fruit allows customization. Tie up in cellophane for a perfect grab-and-go gift.

3. **Jarred 'Nice Cream' Surprise:** Individual mason jars, each with a different blend-in frozen right in it (peanut butter swirl, cocoa nib, mashed berry). Include instructions to top with milk of choice and blend!

4. **Herbal Tea Blends:** Dried fruits, herbs, and spices offer natural sweetness. Include a beautiful infuser to elevate the present!

Additional Considerations

- **Transparency:** Letting the host know what makes your dish diabetes-friendly offers reassurance and can inspire others with healthier choices.

- **Sharing the Knowledge:** If baking a healthier treat, feel free to subtly include the recipe card alongside! It spreads the delicious (and healthier) love far beyond the event.

Notes

- No "Cheating": The term can bring a lot of shame to managing a condition like diabetes. This chapter's focus is on enjoying the occasions and finding delicious ways to balance them.

- Flexibility: These are starting points. Get creative and customize based on personal preference!

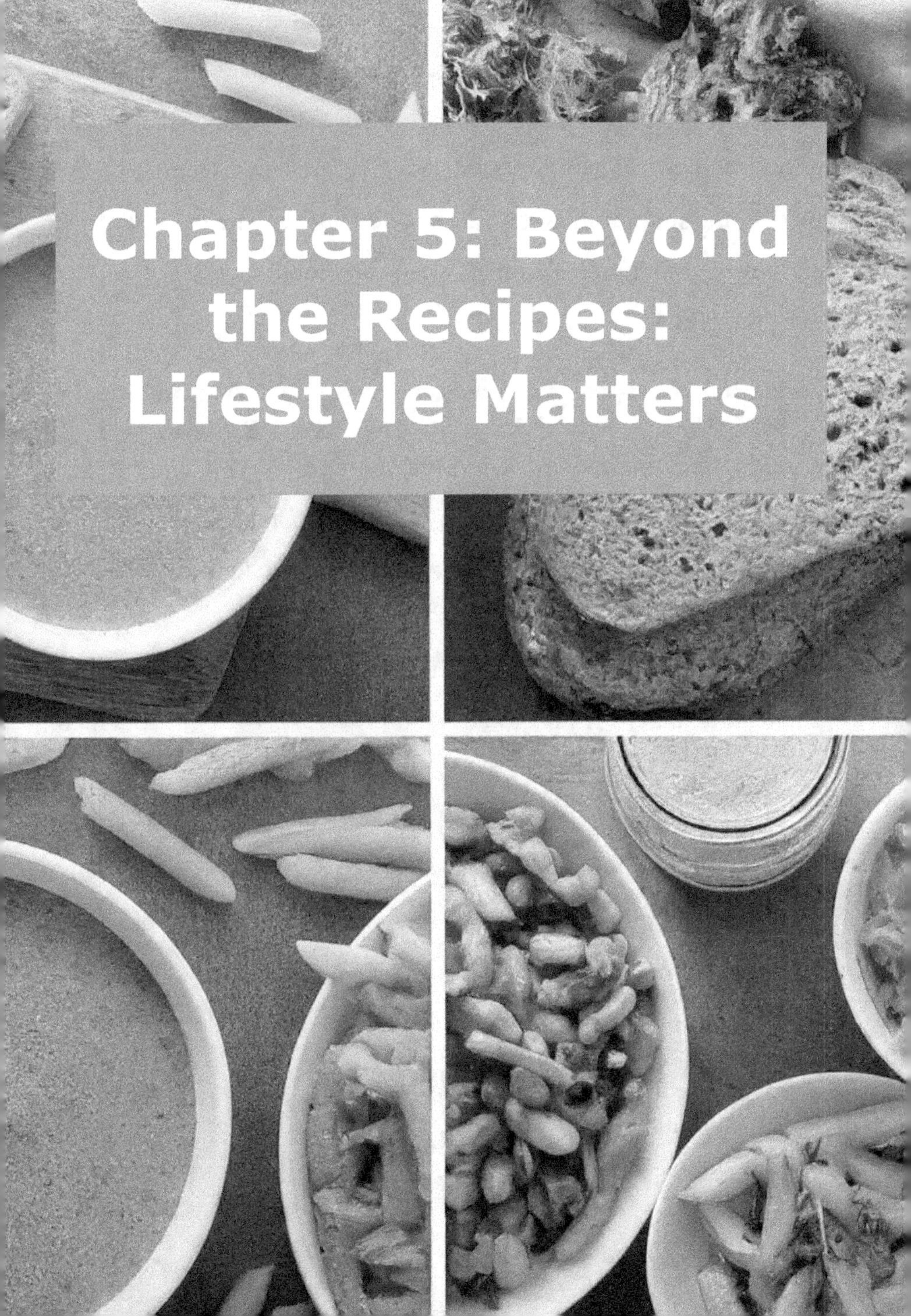
Chapter 5: Beyond
the Recipes:
Lifestyle Matters

It's tempting to jump right into flavors and textures when we think about food. Yet, when managing diabetes, the magic happens in the spaces *between* bites. This chapter isn't about guilt or adding yet another "to-do" – it's about empowerment! Let's uncover the simple shifts that, alongside your tasty new dietary plan, can have a monumental impact on your blood sugars and overall well-being.

Hydration Power: Beyond Basic Thirst

Water is, quite literally, life's foundation. Dehydration, even at mild levels, can play havoc with our blood sugar management. How? It messes with our body's systems, from digestion to hormone balance. *But let's make this joyful, not a chore!*

- **The Flavor Factor:** Get creative with natural water infusions! Think sliced fruit, herbs, even a touch of cucumber for spa-like vibes.

- **Herbal Delights:** A world of unsweetened teas can enhance hydration while delivering healthy plant compounds. From vibrant hibiscus to comforting chamomile, there's a taste for every mood.

- **Sugar Swaps:** If plain water seems daunting, go for naturally flavored, zero-sugar seltzers or a tiny splash of real fruit juice in your water.

Mindful Eating: Rediscovering Your Inner Cues

In our hurry-up world, eating often becomes mindless. Mindful eating isn't a complex practice; it's about reconnecting with the simple joy of nourishment. Let's get practical:

1. **Sensual Focus:** Before every bite, take a moment. Look at the colors, appreciate the aroma, anticipate the first texture as it hits your tongue. Slow down, and satisfaction follows.

2. **Hunger vs. Craving:** Check in with yourself. Is it true hunger (empty stomach, growling) or emotional craving? Both are valid, but mindful eating lets us honor them differently.

3. **The Pause:** After half your portion, take a break. A few minutes give your stomach time to tell your brain, "Hey, I'm getting there!" This stops overeating in its tracks.

The Big Picture: Habits That Hold

Snacks and desserts are fantastic, but true blood sugar success is holistic. Here's how lifestyle boosts your whole journey:

- ✓ **Planning Power:** Even light meal prep makes healthy choices the default, especially at those vulnerable "need food NOW" moments.

- ✓ **Movement Matters:** Every little bit counts! It's not just about calorie burn – exercise also improves your body's sensitivity to insulin. Find something you love, even a brisk walk makes a difference.

✓ **Your Support System:** Diabetes can feel isolating. Lean on those who cheer you on – doctors, loved ones, even online communities. Shared experience is powerful medicine.

From Knowledge to Power

This chapter isn't about perfection. It's about awareness. Small changes, done consistently, create amazing long-term shifts. Don't be afraid to experiment and find what feels truly good and sustainable for *you*. This is your journey to thriving, both on the plate and beyond!

Notes:

- **Encouraging, Not Preachy:** No one needs more food rules. This emphasizes how these fit into a joyful, healthy life.

- **Practicality:** Simple tips to incorporate immediately enhance reader engagement.

- **Focus on Individuality:** Emphasizing that there's no "one-size-fits-all" approach.

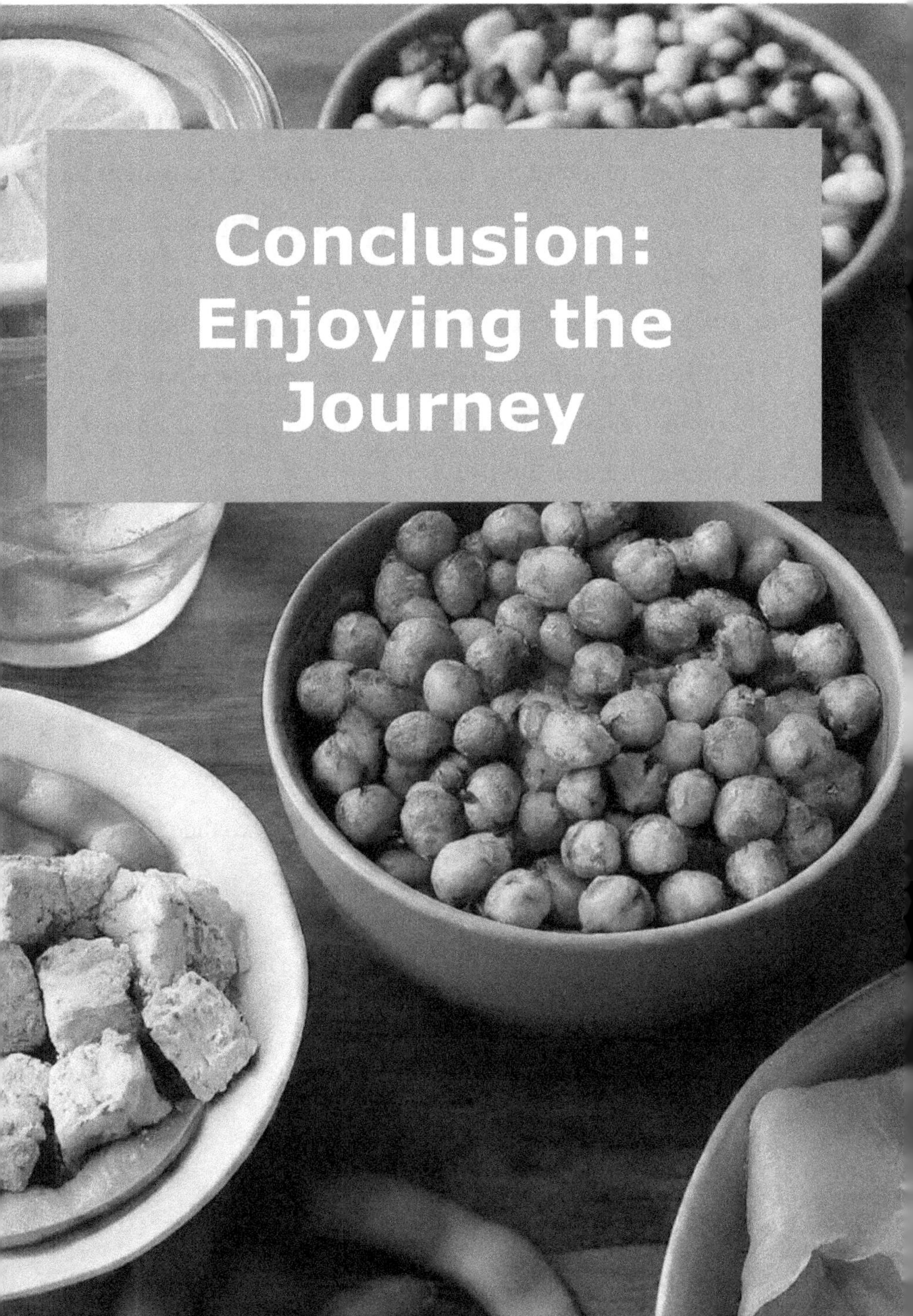

Conclusion: Enjoying the Journey

D iabetes management can feel like an uphill climb at times. That's where the flavors, textures, and satisfaction of these recipes come into play. This book isn't just about controlling your blood sugar; it's about recapturing the delight food can bring to your life! And remember, this isn't a rigid prescription; it's a starting point for exploration.

- **Progress Over Perfection:** Some days will be more on track than others, and that's okay. What matters is consistently coming back to healthy choices and learning from both successes and stumbles.

- **A Culinary Adventure:** Discover new ingredients, play with flavors, and don't be afraid to experiment. Cooking and baking aren't just necessities for those with diabetes - they can become hobbies to cherish!

- **Celebrating Moments:** A vibrant snack that makes a stressful day brighter, a decadent dessert shared with loved ones, these are the sweet points of a balanced life with diabetes.

A Note from Avery

My sincerest hope is that these recipes and all the knowledge packed into this book not only support your diabetic journey but also spark genuine joy in your kitchen. Please, share your creations with me, tell me about your challenges and triumphs! We're a community in this, and celebrating those wins - big and small - makes the journey so much sweeter.

Share Your Voice!

Let me know which recipes are your favorites... and those you think could use a tweak in the next edition! Your feedback helps this book become an even better tool for others along the path of managing diabetes deliciously.

DIABETES MEAL PLAN TRACKER

DIABETES MEAL PLAN

Tracker

1200-CALORIE LOW-CARB DIET PLAN

	protein	carbs	fat	total calories
meals	15% -30%	**40% - 65%**	20%-35%	1200 to 1500 calories

DAILY CALORIES SAMPLE

	protein	**carbs**	**fat**	**total calories**
Mushroom & lentil scramble	20 gm	25 gm	15 gm	350 calories
Tuscan white bean soup with kale & sausage	25 gm	45gm	20 gm	400 calories
Salmon and veggie stir-fry with Quinoa	35 gm	30 gm	20 gm	400 calories
Roasted beet chips	1 gm	8 gm	2 gm	52 calories
total	81 gm	78 gm	57 gm	1202 kcal

DIABETES DIET MONTHLY TRACKER

DIABETES DIET MONTHLY TRACKER | MONTH ____________

date	meal	drink	protein	carbs	fat	cal.
1						
2						
3						
4						
5						
6						
7						
8						
9						
10						
11						
12						
13						
14						
15						
16						
17						
18						
19						
20						
21						
22						
23						
24						
25						
266						
27						
28						
29						
30						
31						

DIABETES DIET MONTHLY TRACKER | MONTH __________

date	meal	drink	protein	carbs	fat	cal.
1						
2						
3						
4						
5						
6						
7						
8						
9						
10						
11						
12						
13						
14						
15						
16						
17						
18						
19						
20						
21						
22						
23						
24						
25						
266						
27						
28						
29						
30						
31						

DIABETES DIET MONTHLY TRACKER | MONTH __________

date	meal	drink	protein	carbs	fat	cal.
1						
2						
3						
4						
5						
6						
7						
8						
9						
10						
11						
12						
13						
14						
15						
16						
17						
18						
19						
20						
21						
22						
23						
24						
25						
266						
27						
28						
29						
30						
31						

DIABETES DIET MONTHLY TRACKER | MONTH __________

date	meal	drink	protein	carbs	fat	cal.
1						
2						
3						
4						
5						
6						
7						
8						
9						
10						
11						
12						
13						
14						
15						
16						
17						
18						
19						
20						
21						
22						
23						
24						
25						
266						
27						
28						
29						
30						
31						

DIABETES DIET MONTHLY TRACKER | MONTH _____________

date	meal	drink	protein	carbs	fat	cal.
1						
2						
3						
4						
5						
6						
7						
8						
9						
10						
11						
12						
13						
14						
15						
16						
17						
18						
19						
20						
21						
22						
23						
24						
25						
266						
27						
28						
29						
30						
31						

DIABETES DIET MONTHLY TRACKER | MONTH _______________

date	meal	drink	protein	carbs	fat	cal.
1						
2						
3						
4						
5						
6						
7						
8						
9						
10						
11						
12						
13						
14						
15						
16						
17						
18						
19						
20						
21						
22						
23						
24						
25						
266						
27						
28						
29						
30						
31						

DIABETES DIET MONTHLY TRACKER | MONTH __________

date	meal	drink	protein	carbs	fat	cal.
1						
2						
3						
4						
5						
6						
7						
8						
9						
10						
11						
12						
13						
14						
15						
16						
17						
18						
19						
20						
21						
22						
23						
24						
25						
266						
27						
28						
29						
30						
31						

DIABETES DIET MONTHLY TRACKER | MONTH ________

date	meal	drink	protein	carbs	fat	cal.
1						
2						
3						
4						
5						
6						
7						
8						
9						
10						
11						
12						
13						
14						
15						
16						
17						
18						
19						
20						
21						
22						
23						
24						
25						
266						
27						
28						
29						
30						
31						

DIABETES DIET MONTHLY TRACKER | MONTH __________

date	meal	drink	protein	carbs	fat	cal.
1						
2						
3						
4						
5						
6						
7						
8						
9						
10						
11						
12						
13						
14						
15						
16						
17						
18						
19						
20						
21						
22						
23						
24						
25						
266						
27						
28						
29						
30						
31						

DIABETES DIET MONTHLY TRACKER | MONTH __________

date	meal	drink	protein	carbs	fat	cal.
1						
2						
3						
4						
5						
6						
7						
8						
9						
10						
11						
12						
13						
14						
15						
16						
17						
18						
19						
20						
21						
22						
23						
24						
25						
266						
27						
28						
29						
30						
31						

DIABETES DIET MONTHLY TRACKER | MONTH __________

date	meal	drink	protein	carbs	fat	cal.
1						
2						
3						
4						
5						
6						
7						
8						
9						
10						
11						
12						
13						
14						
15						
16						
17						
18						
19						
20						
21						
22						
23						
24						
25						
266						
27						
28						
29						
30						
31						

DIABETES DIET MONTHLY TRACKER | MONTH __________

date	meal	drink	protein	carbs	fat	cal.
1						
2						
3						
4						
5						
6						
7						
8						
9						
10						
11						
12						
13						
14						
15						
16						
17						
18						
19						
20						
21						
22						
23						
24						
25						
266						
27						
28						
29						
30						
31						

www.ingramcontent.com/pod-product-compliance
Lightning Source LLC
Chambersburg PA
CBHW050835260726
48660CB00006B/2257